Echoes
From My
heart

Echoes
From My

heart

My words gifted to you
to comfort, guide, inspire

jlKEEZ

Echoes From My Heart:
My words gifted to you to comfort, guide, inspire

National Library of Australia

Cover Illustrator: Sally Jaquet, blaqjaqdesign.com
Formatter: Stephanie Anderson Alt 19 Creative
Author Photo: Dr. Paije Cox

ISBN: 978-0-6488753-4-5 (paperback)
ISBN: 978-0-6488753-5-2(ebook)

1st Edition

In Praise of
Echoes
From My

JL Keez's words capture true emotion and authenticity, giving the reader an inside look and a deep understanding of what it is like to struggle with mental illness. Not only are her words captivating and clearly reflective of pain and struggle but also of thriving and surviving, giving the reader hope! My emotions and thoughts were awakened as I experienced her powerful and very honest words reflected in this gift of beautiful verse.

NELIA HUTT, CEO TRAVEL LIVE GIVE PODCAST, AUTHOR
PHILANTHROPIST AND MENTAL HEALTH ADVOCATE, CANADA

J L has lived a life and a half and has a story to tell which comes straight from the heart in lyrical looping verse. Her words may heal, soothe and inspire you as you travel the road within.

JEMMA RICHARDS, LOVE THIS FOOD THING PODCAST, UK

Insightful, heartfelt and wonderful. A journey of struggle and triumph through verse.

LEE BELPERIO, LAB ASSISTANT AND WELL-BEING SUPPORT
THE DEPARTMENT OF EDUCATION, SOUTH AUSTRALIA

To those who walked beside me as I endured the impact of mental illness, up until its demise. Your contributions, timely in arriving, kept my focus forward and determination strong. Indebted…

Is there a whisper
Calling from within
A quiet echo
Longing for your attention
Your undivided attention
Do not ignore this tiny voice
For this is that part of you
Answering to the call
For explanation

In desperation it nudges
Employing you to stop
In the silence
Listen, hear
Allow the silence to speak
Give the whisper your time
After-all, this is the divine
This is YOU

Reaching from a place
Held in high respect
Longing to commune
Where whispers, and,
The quiet echo
Join in conspired consultation
With your heart
To comfort, guide, inspire you
Out of the suffering

Preface

Where illness lines your days and nights, comfort, guidance and inspiration is deserved in whatever form best suits the individual. As I navigated recovery from a range of mental illnesses—an eating disorder, chronic fatigue, migraines, depersonalisation, OCD and suicidal depression—I sought refuge via a range of avenues.

Raising my children brought distraction and smiles, family pets gave unconditional love and reading inspirational stories and verse often gave me exactly what I needed to hear in a particular moment. This is why, with having written so many verses during my recovery, I have decided to share these with you, plus a range of new ones scribed especially for this book.

Finding myself in the trenches of hopelessness far too often I would reach out for words that would nurture. The power of words being strung together for the purpose of lifting souls who struggle is empowering. Especially where the words shared are written by one who has suffered before you. The wisdom imparted adds a hug when required!

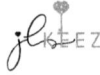

Echoes From My Heart is the gift I give. Each verse is written from my heart space, as I wanted each to resonate, make sense, and contribute meaning for the reader. I find that writing from the heart gives a quality to words only possible through doing so. As you read know each word was felt by me as I gifted it to you.

Reading verse is different to reading a book. Due to their shortness in length, this allows one to surrender to the verse for a brief moment, or stay a little longer should re-reading be required. Each verse stands alone, not relying upon the previous pages, nor needing to prepare you for what is ahead!

Verse gets to the point, takes you on a journey of comfort and leaves you uplifted quickly!

Should you be searching for moments of clarity, direction, or simply words to bring rest when weary, verse may be the valuable addition to your recovery tool kit!

May my verses add solace, a measure of reassurance, and compassion as you navigate and heal the story of your life.

Introduction

For me, verse comes easy. I will be given a line through thought and immediately know all must stop while I write the remainder! Most often I do not know where the verse is taking me until, in conclusion, I re-read. Rarely is a verse drafted for change; it stands as originally written.

This can find me writing many in a day. Subsequently, this may also find me calling out for the words to stop and come back tomorrow!

Verse is one of those privileges we as humans have access to for various purposes. As my collection grew I realised they indeed held purpose. It was my turn to provide a healing thought for those suffering in life; searching for respite. The next step - how do I achieve this?

Well, I simply start a manuscript and see where it ends up! The result, pages of verse, in no particular order, occupying their own space. Some of the verses are quite short, some longer.

Exactly how this book is utilised is up to the reader. You may start at the beginning and take yourself on a day to day journey. You may open at will, read, mark this one off as 'done' and close. Or, you may do the random 'thing' and find yourself revisiting verses often. In this latter scenario I would suggest they must be important, holding value for you at this time in your life. Hold them close. Due to the nature of this book, there is not a 'contents' page as such.

You may develop favourites. Others may not seem to speak to you at all; these you simply let go of. Healing is different for all. We each deserve words that meet our need, but this can be quite varied in nature from one person to another. Hence the inclusion of so many!

What I have come to know, and therefore with confidence propose, whichever verse you open to it will hold relevance for your current life situation. The relevance may be small, or a huge eye-opening moment cascading down on you. Flow with their lead.

I start with the verse '*When a child is Born*'. This one emphasises the conclusion I came to toward the close of my recovery days; the need to allow each soul to be the one they were born to be. I conclude with '*To the tune of the Breeze*'. These beautiful words remind us of the wonder of life and how to enjoy our time while here. I think you will understand why this one when you read it! In between lies a variety of reassurance!

Whether in recovery, searching for answers as to why your body hurts, or simply wishing to enjoy verse, may your time spent here enlighten, deliver understanding, and most of all, comfort, guide and inspire.

When a child is born
Marvel at the beauty
Be intrigued by who they will be
Nurture the needs as they present
Watch for indicators as to what will be defining
characteristics
Attributes, interests, likes, dislikes, personality traits
Get excited that you are the privileged one witnessing this
soul progress
Support the inherent aspects that together complete this
child
Unconditionally accept

Do not demand, scold, condemn, disapprove, criticise
Instead gently show them the way with loving approval
Help them celebrate the uniqueness they represent
Allow them to fall down and learn, their strength will grow
from here
Don't call them naughty ... how do they know?
Guide this child to know

And when the child is all grown up
Be glad you know who they are
Not who you made them be

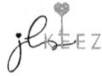

jLKEEZ

Black Seed

The black seed of truth
Holds the power of freedom
The power to release
The power to rejoice

So when this darkness
Emerges from within
Do not escape or run away
Do embrace the meaning shared
For this will bring the peace you yearn

The black seed of truth
Is a friend worth knowing
The friend who at first
Seemed as a foe

The black seed of truth
Opens the door
To the riches,
The colours of life
Once unknown

The 'Another'

As a heart is torn
Broken by another
The owner has a choice
To condemn their life to graveness
Or, in gratitude,
Thank the lessons taught
The learnings now in place
When shared closeness was the path
Grieve
Then, in strength, begin once more
Heart repaired, anew
Bless the 'another'
Wish them well as they journey forward
For without the inclusion of their soul
In combination with yours
Neither could have grown
To reach the riches now enjoyed

© 2014 J.L. Keez

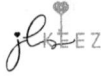

When in fear we do respond
Then it is fear we do create
And hence the cycle goes
Until, in awareness
The cause that drives the fear
Is eliminated, dispelled
Then in love we do respond
And through love we do create

Never Let It Go

When peace has left
Replaced by fear
Where trust has gone
Love disappears

The body wilts
Life dwindles
Saddens

The return to wholeness
Requires the owner
To look within
To find what's missing

The love of self
Will restore the soul
This is the link to all answers sought

Embrace this emotion
Hold it dear
Own its power
Never let it go

In a Sea of Misunderstanding

Standing alone
In a sea of misunderstanding
Waves endlessly roll by
Taking my soul to the depths
Of internal despair

Indignant voices
Using words to denigrate
Sound as sirens in my mind
Reminding me daily
That suffering is a lonely game

A choice for future beckons
Do I stay, or do I leave
The latter convincing
In the debate
Tween survival or depart

The waves grow and swell
Swirling and enticing
Pulling at my body
Engulfing the thoughts
Until they merge as one

Then a voice from somewhere close
Speaks softly as I fall
"Do not give way to waves
Or voices that condemn
Stand strong against the tide"

"For today the pain it beckons
To end beneath the waves
But know tomorrow offers
A hand stretched out
The hand of understanding"

The waves do loose their strength
Subsiding, calming, I stand
The powerful pull weakens
Suicidal thoughts disconnect
The waves retreat

A hand does reach out
The hand of understanding
A voice filled with explanation
Arrives in the nick of time
To inform

Communing with this treasure
Our voices blend in sync
This hand of understanding
Honouring its word
Determined in its resolve

No longer alone
The sea of misunderstanding
Now stilled, waves absent in their pull
The depths of internal despair
Lifts to heights before unknown

Defined by words anew
Shared by the treasure
Where strength abides
Where suicidal thoughts
And waves no longer merge

Standing alone
Has found its end
With gratitude expressed
My turn has now arrived
To share my acquired wisdom

For those who find their days
Standing alone
In a sea of misunderstanding
Where waves and suicidal thoughts
Are dangerously enticing

My hand outstretched
My hand of understanding
Was the purpose of my suffering
To comfort, guide, inspire
Others who suffer too

That choice does exist
Where freedom is the lure

It is in the thinking
The thoughts
Where the debate
Tween survival or depart
Has the power to succeed

You see, your thoughts took you
Into the depths of internal despair
Your thoughts lifted you
To the heights
Where now your strength abides

At the end of the day
The ability to heal
To turn your life around
Was right there in your thoughts
Being guided was required

Your thoughts
That voice from somewhere close
The guided tour undertaken
Via the hand of understanding
Was you all along

Returning you home
You fought the tides
That threatened
Where the choice to exist
Gave you freedom as the lure

© 2022 J.L. Keez

The Story

This is the story I once saw
This is the story I was a part of
This is the story that took my soul
This is the story that broke my spirit

This is the story I choose to leave behind
This is the story whose frame I step away from
This is the story I no longer keep
This is the story I no longer speak

This is the story no longer mine
This is the story that is yours alone
This is the story you came to regret
This is the story you should not have created

For stories like this
Deliver pains so deep
For both story creator and story victim

I relinquish the story
From depths of despair
For this is required for the story...
To fade, disconnect, lose power

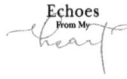

I yield to the peace now dwelling within
Bask in this freedom
As this is the space for ...
A new story to begin

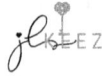

Soul

My soul left the other day
Said it needed to go away
To commune quietly with its internal self
To solve a wondering, unsettling

"But what will people think and say"
A phrase when spoken
Unleashes tears and extreme fears
Anxiety of proportions immense

Upon rejoining me today
The soul speaks the answer
Long term sought
A knowledge of clarity

These words that haunted the soul for years
Were given power over the soul
As abuse inflicted took its blame
Deeply injecting, infusing all cells

In letting go of this false learning
The soul felt free, light, relieved
These feelings soul now handed to me
As once more we joined as one

Another hurdle overcome

The chorus of welcoming sounds
Ring out across the morn

The rays of magnificent sun
Shine radiant upon the earth

The birds in harmonious song
Bring excitement as they fly

The beetles, the bugs do scurry
In search of sustenance for their day

The petals of flowers open
Adding fragrance to the air

The trees wake from quiet slumber
Shaking the nightly yawn from their leaves

And just as nature prepares to welcome us
We in return spread our arms in acceptance

To embrace the events to come
Designed, created to enhance our lives

For this is the purpose of the morning ritual
Where nature and human join in collaboration

To walk the path of life side by side
Where well-being is lined with jubilant bliss

Instead!

They call it blushing!
I call it embarrassing
When taking my turn to speak
But even this messenger
Not at all liked
Conveys that deep longing
To fit in, belong
Afraid of criticism
A strong feature shaping
My developing character
As words I now share
The acknowledging snickers
Serve to reinforce
The distance I feel from others in life

So 'blushing' I need, for you to hear
Please leave my face
You are not welcome here
Return to the place you duly came from
And do not appear again
Your presence for me means loneliness
Is this clear?
Blushing I know your intent is to inform
I get it, understand and know why you surface
But truly my dear
Your services are now obsolete
For I have grown, recognising your purpose
Yes I belong, I do hold a place
In life, I'm important, so you I erase

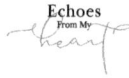

Thanks for the learning, for that I'm indebted
The strength you provided is gratefully accepted
But, not with malice, I say to you now
"The coming and going, not quite knowing when,
Was truly annoying, let's not pretend.
Knowing you are redundant, have gone from my life
The peace now prevailing is welcome relief."

A face holding its natural complexion
While speaking aloud to groups that gather
Or singing to those willing to listen!
Offers the owner, that would be me
Opportunities to share without dreaded fear
To open my mouth in confidence, in acceptance
This I prefer

Instead!

© 2014 J.L. Keez

How to just...
Simply...
Be!

Didn't I sweep you up
Into the dustpan
Put you in the bin

Why then am I feeling you
Underneath my foot
Pushing sharply through
The sole of my shoe

"There remains a piece
Of unearthed worry
Beneath the surface
Of your skin
My role is to remove it"

So, as I ponder the meaning
My mind wonders to a fear
Lodged firmly in my heart
If I be me...is that OK
What can I do
What can't I do

"Although this fear has shown itself
On occasions throughout the years
And we have wrestled with
Answers presenting for consideration
There lingers uncertainty
A lack of surety
This is why I found your sole"

Knowing this unsettledness
Has continued like a thread
The moment has arrived
To solve it and move on
So in meditative solitude
I ask once more to know
What can I do, what can't I do
When wellness turns up for me

"To know the response
Sit quietly some more
Clear your mind to clarity
To hear the words sentenced just for you
And when the words appear
Spoken softly to your soul
Know they travel safely
From that place within
That represents your truth"

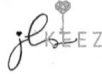

"Just live within each moment
As life unfolds each day
Listen intently to your body
For this will be your guide
Of what can be, of what can't be
And as trust builds in listening
This practise soon will bring
The comfort, the tranquillity
The insurance that you seek
Of how to live authentically"

In considered response
I now take theses words
And live by them each day
And just like that
Each moment lived
Does show me the way
What I can do, what I can't do
Clearly speaks to me
In freedom I have found peace
In now knowing, understanding ...

How to just ...
Simply ...
Be!

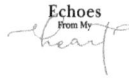

Release the negative
As positivity
And all its peace
Lives here

It is how we respond to a life event
As to whether it is deemed
Cruel, or
Just a beautiful lesson
Sent to enrich our lives
Whilst here

jLkEEZ

And there I *see* ...

I look through the window
And there I see me
A reflection of anguish
Looking back at me

I look through the window
And there I see glimpses
Flashbacks from my life
Looking back at me

I look through the window
And there I see you
Struggling to speak
Looking back at me

I look through the window
And there I see many
Offering opinions
Looking back at me

I look through the window
And there I see loneliness
Bleak and so sad
Looking back at me

I look through the window
And there I see you ... again
This time with strength, speaking freely, firmly
Looking back at me

I look through the window
And there I see me ... again
Grateful for the words you conveyed
Looking back at me

I look through the window
And there I see colour replace bleak
The sad has left, gone with bleak
Looking back at me

I look through the window
And there I see peace
Surrounding me, filling me
Looking back at me

I look through the window
And there I see the purpose of seeing
Me, flashbacks, you, many, loneliness
You, me, colour and peace

The window was sent
To communicate the path
Taken over the years
To show me I've endured, survived, won

Looking back at me ...

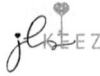

But who was the you
Struggling to speak
Then in time gaining strength
Looking back at me

This was the voice
Locked away at first
Scared to share insights
Looking back at me

This was the true self
Hidden from view, remaining quiet
Until in healing had come forth
Looking back at me

So now as...

I look through the window
And now I see me
This is the whole me
Yes, me and you

Looking back at me...

Shadows and Shades

As the shadows of my life
Show themselves to me
The shades come out in force
To protect my questioning mind

As the shadows grow in volume
The shades begin to fade
For the shadows are fully aware
As are the shades
That although once purposeful
So needed in their roles
They now hinder the path to healings truths

With the collection of shadows explained
Their content and affect
They loose their place, their power
Their attachments to my soul

My mind finds peace
From examining shadows long list
The shades can now retire and rest
From years of protective living
Confident that as shadows, and as shades
They have each concluded their roles in my life
A life once filled with seemingly endless, nameless pains

jl Keez

As life now transforms

I give thanks to the voices, the wisdoms
The caring natures of...

Shadows and Shades

When lives cross paths
A greater purpose unfolds
For the connection
Created in collaboration
Between mind, spirit, body and soul
Has arrived just on time
To deliver the lessons
The learnings required
For each to heal, to grow, transcend
And whether the connection
Is long or short
Know the importance for each
Will last throughout this life
And those yet to come

© 2015 J.L. Keez

jLKEEZ

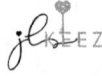

Dreams are the birthstone of life
Filling nights with anticipation
Days with contemplated wonderings

The place where each collide
Is when the dreams of intuition
Meet the realities of daily existence

In excited renditions
The synchronicity of day
Delivers the visions of night

This is when, in acknowledgement
We know, our story is unfolding
As divinely scribed

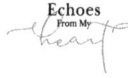

Breathe

As the light of day spreads its warmth
Breathe in the glow
For this is a gift for you
Free in its delivery
To invigorate, inspire, intoxicate
Nurture and nourish
So your day ahead
Fills with all that is deserved

Simply breathe

jLkeez

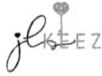

Register that demeanour you wear today
Is it uplifting
Or deprecating
Should it be the latter
May I encourage you to stop
For a moment
Take a deep breath
And start again!

Embrace the positive
Leave deprecating in the nearby bin!

Bouquet and Intrigue

Life is a wonderful bouquet of flowers
A tapestry of intrigue
Filled with an expanse of colour
An array of possible experiences

But do select your blooms wisely
And tapestry with care

For each has the ability
To enhance, or lead astray
Hold yourself close
As you decide

Ensure the blooms
The tapestry
Reflects the truth
Of who, and how, you wish to be

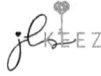

jl KEEZ

Colours

If your life is shrouded in grey
Then, in your mind
Pick up that paint brush
Add the colours desired
Visualise wearing these colours
Feel the colours
Behave the colours
Think the colours

In mindful presentation
Watch your life explode
Where colour illuminates
And grey

Has no place to reside

© 2021 J.L. Keez

The Calm

Deep within the soul resides the calm
Yes, that is the voice you hear
In the silence of the night
Which at the moment is ignored
Heard as words simply appearing in your thoughts
Seemingly made up

But from this time forward
If I may, listen with intent
For that voice is your best friend
Connecting through the dark
Inviting you to commune
Deep within the soul where
...your calm summons, awaits

© 2021 J.L. Keez

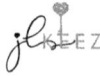

Are You Ready

As the curtains are opened
And the sun joins your day
Acknowledge the sounds, be
Aware of the magic
About to enter your life

For this is what's on offer
Fun, Frivolity
Fantastic experiences
Fortified with explosions of colour
Filled with treasured moments

A whole lot of magic

Are you ready...

As the rain clears
The mist departs
Rainbows of colour
Shine through the haze
Beckoning

As the step is taken
To go beyond the confine
One realises
Understands

That the once boundary
Of imposed darkness
Represented through tears
Has found its end
For colour has returned

Infusing its message
Of hope, tranquility
Of peace, of triumph
Of healing

You are now ready
To live, to thrive
For this was the purpose
Of darkness
To deliver the colour

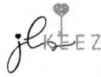

When, in readiness
Acceptance of self
Transformed, transcended
The one once lost

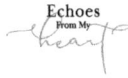

Diamond

The most treasured diamond
Is not the one you wear
Nor the one you hope for
It is the one residing within
The authentic unrivalled soul
You have the privilege of calling
YOU

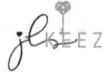

Home

The morning dew
Feels like bursts of joy
As my feet
Connect

Looking up I see
Blooms of flowers
And the leaves of trees
Opening

My heart responds
With a rush of triumph
An openness of
Love

The morning sun
Baths my soul
The 'connect', the 'opening', the 'love'
Liberating

Arms outstretched
The warmth of day infuses
The smile worn, tells me, I am

Home

'Unrehearsed' to 'Rehearsed'

Unrehearsed and ready to live
The stage we stand upon
May waver, may still
We stutter, we fall
We climb, we navigate
It is in being
'Unrehearsed'
Where excitement may join us
Or trepidation linger
But do know this
Life is of your making
And as the days
And nights pass
'Unrehearsed'
Will turn its attention
To the growth
From wisdom acquired
As life is lived
It is when we move from
'Unrehearsed' to 'Rehearsed'
That the maturity of experience
Sees us rise to our calling
Our life's purpose
Where the wobbliness
Of those days
And nights
Spent in 'unrehearsing'

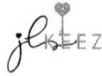

Prepared us for the strength
Of...
'Rehearsed'

Kettle and Steam

Steam explodes from the kettle
Imposing its presence upon the wall
Leaving its mark
A glistening shine
Felt as heat

It is as though
The kettle upon waking
Felt issue with the morn
And took upon itself
To express this through steam

The wall did not complain
For it had wondered when
The kettle would explode
For it had witnessed
Its pain for years

In turning to the kettle
It smiled from behind the paint
That kind of smile
That says,
"At last!"

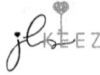

So if you are like the kettle
Wanting to express your pain
Through anger
Or some sort of explosion
Please do!

But once decided
Do consider those around you
Choose your target wisely
The one who understands
Supports

Not the one aloof
Nor the one lacking empathy
For you deserve to be acknowledged
And given the space
To release

To heal

I walk into my presence
And what do I see
I see joy, at last
Where once sorrow stood
I see smiles, at last
Where once tears fell
This is the presence of love
The emotion now felt
As days of suffering
Depart

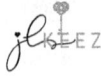

jLkeez

The Sun

Have you ever wondered
Why the sun is yellow
And filled with warmth

Well,
I think it has something to do
With its caring role

Of being that
Well-worn yellow blanket
Spreading its glow

For each of us
To feel, and know
We are loved

This is the purpose
The reason
Why yellow

Is the colour of choice

Echoes
From My
heart

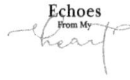

Stretched before us
Every day
Is the platter of life
Enticing, yet cautionary

Adopt wiseness in selection
Diligence when experiencing
For each of your selections
Determine life ahead

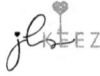

jLkEEz

You *see*

You see my pain
But do not *feel* my pain
You see my angst
But do *feel* my angst
You see my suffering
But do not *feel* my suffering

For without experience
My life is a complete unknown
For without empathy
My life is but a nothing
For without knowledge
My life is misunderstood

Do not judge what you do not know
Do not speak words which do not help
Do not side line my life
For in doing so
You null and void my truth
You dismiss without consideration
You take away ... me

A Whisper of Wind

Captured in the moment
A whisper of wind
Echoes a message
Heaven sent
"Do not despair
Nor fold under the weight,
For today a revelation
A truth
Will find its way to you"

And just as promised
The truth did find its way
"You are believed
You are not crazy
The card life dealt you
Is not so easy
But in strength
You will prevail"

Lifted, renewed
That whisper of wind
Echoed once more
"Your strength is now you own"
Captured in the moment

What a blessing

When the ground opens
To seemingly swallow
Strengthen within
As much as you can
For this is the time
To go even deeper
To resolve those lingering
Doubts
Those lingering moments
Held in thought

Endure the days of impossible pain
Grieve the time when
Life took your soul
Work hard to understand
Create a new frame for your story
And when, in truth
You realise you were right all along
Rejoice

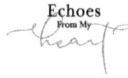

Then in gratitude
Give thanks to this time
Although painful in its delivery
It has given you the greatest of gifts
Final freedom from the choices of others
A strength, an understanding
Able to be shared with those
Who suffer the same

... What a blessing ...

The Broken Record of Time

The broken record of time
Is like a never ending cycle
Circling to jolt, to awaken
Events held in memory
Impacting the view of the world

As scratches form
From repeated visits
Events likeminded in content
Cry out in pain
"Please hear my words"

'This cycling will not conclude
Until in exploration
The purpose is found
There is healing required
Take heed and hear"

For in doing so
The events held in memory
Will find their demise
The circling will cease
The never ending cycle end

The broken record of time

It's purpose ... served

Dawn of Time

Since the 'dawn of time'
Men who have suffered
Women, classified as delicate
Have met their end
At the hands of misunderstanding

Mental health undiagnosed
Meant suffering endured
Mental health undiagnosed
Meant delicate was lost to ignorance

Over time brave people challenged
Asking the, "Why"
In educated collaboration
Lines of enquiry found solutions
Now on offer for those willing to listen

Mental health now diagnosed
Means the suffering, the delicate
Mental health now diagnosed
Means understanding meets these souls

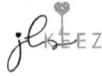

Since the 'dawn of time'
Has experienced a revolt
Where, in moving forward, society
Has available, revolutionary understanding
Giving a new meaning

To the 'dawn of time'

As the book of life
Opens its pages
Scrutinise the dialogue
Scan the photos
Take from each leaf
Those experiences
You know will enhance
Close tight the pages
You know will
Not serve you well

Make each moment count

So when the time arrives
To review your book of life
The pages will tell
Of wonder, of joy
Of a story you made
Your own

Make today a page
Worthy of inclusion

jlkeez

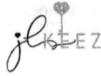

To those who rob your integrity
To those who dismiss your worth

Bid each adieu
Goodbye

For their inclusion in your day
For their place in your life

Has found both its purpose
And its end

Echoes From My Heart

Permission

The process for permission
Has found its way to you
Explore this notion
Is there a space deep within
Holding itself to ransom
Unable to allow the self
The freedom to be

Should this resonate today
Seek to discover the 'why'
Know that the permission deserved
Is pressing you to respond
Give it respect
Your acknowledgement
For the time has arrived

To claim your right
To freely live in peace

Permission will make this so

© 2021 J.L. Keez

57

Thoughts

Are you allowing the future
To bury you alive
Where your mind in worry
Desperate to avoid
Outcomes feared
Is frantically pessimistic

Then, if I may
Let your mind find peace
For tomorrow results
From the thoughts
Created in concern
Today

Redesign the thoughts
Visualise a tomorrow
Free of fear
For this will then
Surely deliver
A future

Where tranquility and calm
Coexist in harmony

Downfall

When your downfall
Becomes
Your greatest strength
You know
The purpose of the
Suffering
Has found its Waterloo!

You are now ready
Equipped
To face, design
A life
So wonderful
Tempered through the
Knowledge gained

When the downfall
Took your soul
Twisted it in knots
Caused tears
And even tantrums
Before
In resolution

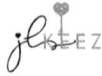

You now hold
The greatest teacher
In your hands
A wealth of understanding
Of why you were
As now you live
Each waking day

Who you truly are...

Little Bird

I see you
I hear you
I wish I was like you

Your bright tuneful chirp
Brings a smile to my face
Without a care in the world
You happily skip
From branch to branch
Scouring for food
Or is that morsels
To prepare a home for newborns
What ever your purpose
Know you have brightened my morn
Reminding me
That life can be a pleasure
A simple fact of existence
Where unnecessary impacts
Need not exist

And just like that
A random act of kindness
As you fly a little left
To aid another
In search of their morning morsels
Before returning in harmony
To the endeavours
Guiding your morn

As humans
We can learn a lot from you
To wake each day
To sing each day
To embrace simplicity
Instead of burying
Our thoughts
In unnecessary quarrel
Causing so much pain

Little one
I see you
I hear you
I strive each day
To be like you

In gratitude
Thank you for the reminder
Of how we all can be
So harmony is our life
Where simplicity is the framework
And kindness the foundation

Imagine and Immerse

As your day opens
Imagine the wings
Of a beautiful butterfly
Spreading wide
In relaxed acknowledgement
Of itself
It's beauty

Hold the vision
In your eyes
Your heart
Your mind
Your body
Emotions and soul

Capture this moment
Infuse, immerse, rejoice
As the visualisation
Instils
Fills

jLkeez

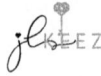

Take this moment with you
Hold it ever so close
Carry it with pride
For this will be
The beauty
You will then
In relaxed acceptance
Radiate
For others to enjoy

In combined acceptance
Allow the practice of
Imagine and immerse
To be a guiding force
As in recovery
You take your life
From suffering
To thriving
So life is once again
A wonder of excitement
Where your future
Reflects your designed

Imagine and immerse

A Hug!

A hug is a warmth shared
A beautiful gesture
A glow in someone's day

Where the message conveyed
Where the emotion given
Where the words unspoken

Speak volumes

Reach out and give a hug
Reach out and receive a hug
Reach inward and give a hug

Today!

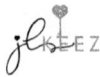

As that tear falls
Collect its wisdom
Hold it for a moment
Allow it to guide
To free you

Then just as quickly
Let it go ...

The Choice

I slipped up in a puddle of mud today
Two choices lie before me
Cry, blaspheme, be angry
Or, in acceptance laugh

For how often do I get
To be a child again
So here I was splashing around
Being free to express
My joy

Then I realised
This is how we all need to live
Free, alive, unrestricted
Accepting all that comes our way

For in doing so
We release our so called burdens
Those thoughts that weigh us down
To view each experience
As a learning regarding life

And how to really
Honestly
Just
Simply be

Emojis and Your Story

Emojis joined our world
When in explanation
Extra embellishment was required

Well though some thought

As the expressions awarded
Grew, multiplied, got crazy
The extent of representation

Brought smiles

As you encounter your life's path
May I suggest
Especially where you are healing

Design your life through emojis

Use these expressions only
Capture your thoughts,
Behaviours, emotions

And when in recovered mode

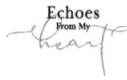

You awake to peace at last
Create that final line
You, love and gratitude

A smile, a heart, a prayer

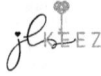

A smile is a measure
The heart does design

A smile is a measure
The answer to a prayer

A smile is a measure
The beginning of a new time

A smile is a measure
The healing is complete

A smile tells its owner
The moment of recovery ensues

A smile tells its owner
The suffering has drawn to a close

A smile tells its owner
The longed for life awaits

A smile tells its owner
The freedom to exist invites

A smile is a measure
A smile tells its owner

You are home ...

The Switch

As the switch of life
Oscillates
Maintain focus
Determination
To weather the downs
Enjoy the ups

Learn from each
For the day
Will arrive
Where the downs
Lessen
The ups, gain momentum

Until in resolution
The downs no longer
Drag, the ups
Refuse to budge
And pesky
Oscillation

jLkeez

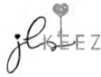

In acknowledged
Acceptance
Gives thanks
That the dizzy days
Of indecision
Have set this intruder

Free ...

© 2021 J.L. Keez

One Day ...

Where words spoken
Are trivial attempts
To close gaps of misunderstanding

Where words spoken
Are empty of meaning
Disguised in embellished jargon

Do acknowledge this is the case
See the reasoning for each
As an inability to own responsibility

Do acknowledge this is the case
See the purpose as a token gesture
From one who cannot do anymore

Then grow in strength
Against the frivolity

Then grow in strength
Against the abandonment

For this was the goal
Of this charade

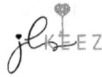

For this was the goal
Of the role you played

To learn the lesson of strength
To take this with you
As your life unfolds
And should thoughts of injustice
Find their way to you once more
Let them go
This was your time to grow
No theirs

Perhaps one day...

Mmmmmm

In a world where authenticity
Has lost its meaning
Where truth has been
Replaced by dare
And women rival men
For equalled positioning

Have you ever thought
This is what illness
Derived from a belief
That self is not enough
Looks like
Particularly mental health

Then try this on for size
A thought to resonate
"Trying to be a man
Is a waste of a woman"
Or in regards to illness
"Trying to not be self
Is a waste of a beauty"

Mmmmmm...

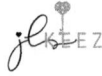

Possibility

Now just what do we mean

Possibility

A chance to grow

Possibility

An alternate road

Possibility

Anything but what is now

Well, maybe...

Possibility

Is the range of wonderful
Choices
Spread before you
To experience
To call your own

Possibility

Is where strength
Meets weakness
For in every decision
Life presents to you
The one selected

Possibility

May enhance
Or destroy...
Honouring the self
Choosing you
Will surely ensure

Possibility

Is exactly where
You need to be
So the life unfolding
Explodes, bringing forth
An expanse of deserved

Possibility

The Frame

Gnarled
Warped
Twisted
The frame worn
Reflects the trauma
Responsible for the shaping
Carried through tears

This frame emerging
From years of disillusionment
Forces the body to yell out
In pain

Explore this frame
Identify the elements
Mal-aligned, disproportionate
Unable to hold together
Support

Pull that frame apart
Ditch the impacting nails
Renovate, rebuild
Design a frame of worth

One bejewelled
Glittering, sparkling
Held together with pride
Where the carried tears release
Allowing a new frame

Steeped in strength
Smoothed through transition
Solid in transcending

To join you
Through your day
Filling you with confidence
That this frame
The result of healing
Will be the pillar of grace
Underlining a life now

Your own…

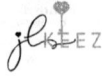

Make your life today
A symbol
Of worth, of excellence
Born of the you
You proudly exhibit
The you proudly called
... Me!

I Wish for You

Of all the wishes hoped this day
I wish for you
A day filled with 'sunshine
Lollypops and rainbows'
A day where life delivers
The greatest of gifts
The wonderment, the awe
Of understanding
That of all the people
Living life today
You are the one most remarkable
The one who has beaten the odds

You stayed
You fought
You recovered
You rose from the depth
Of incredible fear
To emerge triumphant
Ready to fulfil
The wishes, the hopes
Given birth through thought
As each day you battled
To conquer
What you were once told

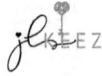

You would never be able to do

But hey, you did ...

Red Wine and Blur

Through the blur of red wine
A haze of crimson hues
Reflections of long held tensions
Appear

Is this an imagined image
Or a truth divine
Beckoning for attention
Coaxing

Immerse within the portrait
Breathe in the meaning depicted
Bath in the emotions felt
Converge

For even though
Intoxication may have
Brought this depiction forth for
Viewing

Somewhere within
Your voice did question
Hence, this is the answer to your
Call

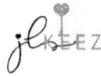

Timely in its delivery
Informative in its care
Take heed, for the time for healing has
Arrived

Capture the visions
Shared in this moment
And when the impact of wine
Retreats

Revisit the reflections
Held in tension
Disperse the hazy crimson
Hues

Then, as healing emanates
Blink those blurs away
Lift above the red wines
Offerings

Recover ...

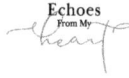

Capturing the essence of you
Is like turning a bright light on
You shine, you glow, you glimmer

You radiate pure joy
Take this you into your day
Today, tomorrow
Everyday!

The power of you

The power of you

The power of you

Take this with you

Wherever you go!

The Thickness of Glass

That prison of fear
Actually made of glass
May be smashed
At any time

However, and don't I know
That glass, although thin
Is as thick as the depth
Of fear carried

One fear at a time
Identified, faced, conquered
Will see the glass
Transform

Dwindling in its depth,
Its seemingly tough domination
Breaking open
Until in freedom

The once held fears
Hold no power
And that glass
Is replaced by

Echoes
From My
heart

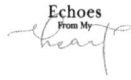

A soft, flexible exterior
Strong in its application
Yet kind in its
Delivery

Where the prison of fear
Gave way
To the pressure exerted
Through ... you got it ...

Smashing!

© 2021 J.L. Keez

Deniability and Plausible

Deniability is one of those choices
Plausible to the owner
A frustration, infuriation
To the receiver

You see,
Where acts of abuse
Accompanied by refutation
Clutched in words of dismissal
Are side-stepped in ownership
A void of loneliness opens for victims

Impacted, left to pick up the pieces
Drooped and wilted, these are the ones
Drifting forward into twisted lives
Characterised by exasperation

Hang on,
Let's define that more clearly
Characterised by sheer utter
Outrage, vexation, rage
Their boundary of protection
Obliterated

This is the realisation demanded
Of those choosing deniability
Clutching to the straws of plausibility
Snubbing the resulting loneliness

To own your actions of refutation
To own your words of dismissal
To go deep within, experience the pain
You inflicted
And when you are entirely ready
... No ... *sorry* is nowhere near enough

Fall to your knees
Outstretch your hands
Drop tears in acknowledgment of the suffering
Overturn the loneliness
Your selfishness did cause

Your display of truths, hurts inflicted
Are deserved admissions of ownership
Given to the victims
Where deniability accompanied by plausibility
Has no place to reside ...

jCkEEZ

Enigmas

Poetry can be an enigma
A beauty to behold
Yet mysterious in its meaning

People can be an enigma
Beauties to behold
Yet mysterious in their expression

This is why preservation
Of the enigmatic notion
Assigned to each at birth

Is encouraged to remain
To be a little perplexing
Where a little bewilderment exists!

For this is where the beauty
The tapestry for life
Will find its magic

In the great expanse of variation
Not in the walls of confinement
Where words conveyed judge

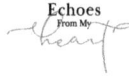

So if today you struggle
With the enigma of you
Throw those thoughts of condemnation

Into the nearest bin
Place a heavy handed lid
Upon the associated words

For we wish to only know
To meet, experience
The enigmatic beauty

Assigned to you ... at birth

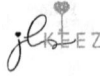

Where the hands of time
Reach out in beckoned form
Their undivided intent
To hand to you
Those answers
When in questioning you cried
"Why do I hurt so much,
Why does my body fold?"

May I gently encourage
You reach back
In connected unification
For together
The healed life desired
Whilst living through pain
Is the shared ideal
Pictured by you, and
The hands of time

Own

Own that ground you stand on
Pull back that veil of doubt
No ... rip it back!

Be obstinate

For there is no one else alive
Who emanates the flow
Of exquisiteness

You project

So own that ground you stand on
Give meaning to your soul
So as that veil dissipates

That ground, your soul
In combined revelation
Shares with us all
The greatness, uniqueness
Of a person worthy of

Existence

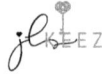

Trees

Trees oxygenate the planet
They generously give life
The act of breathing
Makes this so

But just as intriguing
Trees, like humans
Hold strengths
And weaknesses

Defined by characteristics
Trees fall into categories
Similarly given definition
To human lives

Trees, therefore
Provide a range of metaphors
Ready to apply
To healing journeys across our globe

So here we go ...

Recovery journeys
Tip one from definition to definition
The ultimate goal
To discover the true self
And the definition sought!

Along the way
We see-saw from
Strength to weakness
Being sweet, to being sour
Hoping to end up intelligent
Fearful of being a nerd
Hardening against the strain
Falling to the ground
When it all gets too much
Developing resilience
Surviving pitfalls along the road
We yearn for being the beauty
The unusual, unique

We simply wish to find ourselves
Free of judgement, free of pain
Emerging triumphantly
Where the self stands strong
Against the tides of life
Equipped with a measure
Of self awareness
Born from all the hard work
Recovery demanded

We wane, we falter
We eventually stand strong ...

At first
The Magnolia
Sees us fall to the ground
The weakness winning

Then we morph into
The Sourwood
Disgruntled, angry
Where life tastes so bitter

Next we become
The Dragon Blood
Unusual in its presentation
Dominating our inner desire

In the phase of pleasing
The Sugar Maple
Appears, where we feel the over-riding
Need to sweeten for acceptance

Deciding intelligence is required
The Dodder
Reveals the next unfolding
Perhaps this is who I am

In tired recognition
The Magnolia
Returns
Unable to continue

A deep breath is taken
The Native Palm
Resilient, tough
Lifts the wilted soul

Determined to succeed
The Sycamore
Hard in its awakening
Provides the backbone required

Understanding the necessity
The Noble Fir
Adds its branches of strength
As all areas of healing are addressed

The end of this journey in sight
The River Birch
Urges this survivor
To follow its lead

With a gasp of realisation
The Rainbow Eucalyptus
Demonstrates its rare beauty
In support of the one now so close

The years of searching enveloping
The Balsa Tree
Stands strong
This is the conclusion

Once sought when
The Magnolia
Falling down
In weakness

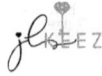

Cried out to
The Balsa
To please return
For I wish to know myself

This is where jubilation is found...

But do understand
That although
The Balsa
Was the ultimate goal
It is the understanding collection
The characteristics
Of each presenting tree
That in combined confession
Will oxygenate
Give life
To the one now standing strong
The act of breathing

Makes this so...

As darkness clears
Shades move to the side
Shadows reveal their truth
Light enters,
The path of life
Now frees
To live
Express
And simply be!

Curve Balls

Life is a wonder
Of magnificent curve balls
Thrown in your direction

Just as one ball
Seems to have found its
Conclusion

Another swings your way
Ready to challenge
To lift you

To the kiddy heights
Of progression
Where nostalgia turns the key

For it is the nostalgic
Returning
In thought only

That sets the stage
Where the heights
Of progression

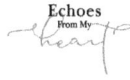

Find their foundation
Their framework
For building

A life anew
Where curve balls
Magnificent in their construction

Take you to the place
Where life is filled with
And reflects

The essence
The purity
The wisdom

The beauty of uniqueness
Only curve balls
Can deliver

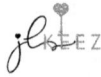

Dear One

Open your eyes
Dear one
Look deep within your soul
Dear one
Bring honesty
Dear one
For here, in clarity
Dear one
Is the wonder
Dear one
The brightness
Dear one
Of a truly genuine soul
Dear one
Yes,
Dear one
I refer
Dear one
To you!

Captured within the muscles
Held as tension
Loud in its expression
Lies the nature
Of the illness
Long term in its affliction

Here-in lies the destination
The mind does need to visit
Should that which lies encased
Give rise to its release
For tension to let go
Recovery ... the reward

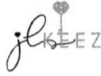

Ignorance

Felt as a splinter
Piercing the brain
The excruciating pain
A messenger
Pay heed to its call
Be discerning in acknowledgment
Most importantly
Do not avoid

Your brain holds your story
The pain reflects the content
This splinter
The indicator

Effectuate a solution
Ignorance is not bliss
Connected consultation
The compulsion required

The puzzle of the mind
Is a mystery to the soul
Until in combined revelation
The secrets, the wanderings
Resolve
And set the spirit free

Mind and the Soul

Where the mind tricks the soul
To believe in a truth
The mind is actually the victim
Not the soul

Yet it is the soul
Which seemingly suffers
Alone
The soul whose tasked

To set itself free
From the cruelty
Of minds games
The mistruths

Yet the soul will learn
As the path toward
Freedom
Is walked

That, sadly, the mind
Is held to ransom
To the stories
It is told

As it was the mind,
Assigned
To guide the soul
Through life

It can only do its best
For no one is sent
To show the mind
Just how to be

So as the soul addresses
Healing each day
Where mistruths eventually
Find their demise

Compassionately sigh
For the mind
Seeming to be
The baddy in all of this

As the victim
Holding your story
It was suffering too
Being pushed and pulled

Until the intelligence
Of the soul
Expert in its application
Frees not only itself

But also the very one
Held ransom to the stories
You actually gave it
To hold

Compassion
Understanding
A hand extended
Will see the soul and mind

Reunite in appreciation
That each was given to the other
To provide comfort
As life took shape, as life took hold

Each was affectively appointed
The role they played
So when the healing of stories
Was asked

The intelligence of the soul
Could work together with the mind
To identify their meaning
Where in collaboration

The mind, the soul
Once more may
Travel through life
As one ...

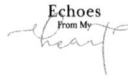

Be the visitor to your childhood
On behalf of your soul
Go where you need to go
To discover the mystery to your illness

For embedded deep within your story
Lies the answers truly sought
You owe your soul, your illness this
To set each free from pain

Maze, Twists, Turns

Life is a wonderful maze
Where twists and turns do dwell
At first a constant exploration
Tempered by those sent to guide

As life unfolds
The twists of fate, the turns then trodden
Begin to question the explorations
Tempered by the hand that guides

The actions lived
Where twists do hurt and turns threaten
Result in cries for explorations to be curbed
Tempered by the voice that guides

Emotions baffled
Twists and turns, twist and turn
Until the explorations undertaken
Tempered by the arm that holds

Find a crossroad
Twists get twisted, the turns lost
Explorations maze fills with haltering
Tempered by the eyes that stare

Echoes
From My
heart

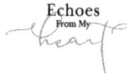

Desperate for understanding
Twists then turn and turns then twist
Until in exhausted exploration
Tempered by the messages taught

The one once filled with fascination
Where twists excited and turns thrilled
When exploration was a joyful living
Tempered by the one now feared

Sees time arrive where the maze of wonder
The twists now confused, and turns now broken
Require new exploration, new direction
Tempered by a voice no longer the misguiding one

Detaching is the key
Where twists untwist, turns repair
New messages to live by formed
Tempered by the one lost all those years

Interrogation of a life once defined by
Twists of trauma and turns of abuse
At last becomes a magnificent maze once more
Tempered by the words of healed revelation

I went to the end of the rainbow
But gold I did not find
Instead, in pure wonder
The most majestic gift
Awaited

Upon closer examination
In awe of this find
I discovered an answer
Long held within my mind

"Who am I,
The one who once shone
Where did I go"

There, dazzling
Was the one I lost so long ago

I picked me up

The fit, exquisite

Shine, or Fade

The sun forgot to shine today
I decided to ask it why
In response the sun did smile

"Like you my friend
Each day we encounter
Is a mix of emotions
Some filled with laughter
Others with pain
And in response
We either shine, or fade"

But aren't you always
Up for a shine
For is that not your job

"Are *you* not always
Up for a shine
Is that not *your* job"
The sun spoke with a smile
"Or do you encounter days
Where your shine
Is lost to a fade"

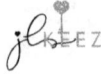

Oh! I said I get it now
Just like me
Your emotions reflect your shine

"Yes dear human
For don't you also see
That each of us who feel
Will shine some days
And fade on others
In reflection to life's
Demands"

Upon reflection
And now with understanding
I replied in the affirmative

"May I add an extra word
For understanding to be complete
Where one encounters
Another without their shine
Do not question the demeanour
Simply be there, supportive
By their side"

In wiseness I now see
The sun and I are no different
To each of us who live

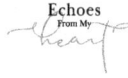

A measure of kindness
Is like a measure of honey

A gesture filled with sweetness
Yet felt for days to come

Whisper

The whisper did whisper
Quiet, yet strong
Please listen with intent
For the meaning I share
As this day unfolds
And you become aware
Hold close to your heart
Your truths and your ways
For this is your grace
The beauty you are
Do not forsake it
But in justice
Take heart
As in truth you live

"But *Life* Got in the Way!"

In the silence I can hear
The loudness of the words
Reaching deep within my soul
Pulling largely at my heart
Words of focused compassion
Screaming out to me

In frustration I did yell
"But life got in the way!"

The words they fell to silence
The chasm of void grew wide
And when I wrongly thought
That my freedom from within
Had found its place at last
The words in disgust returned

"Your body aches each day
Your emotions are all astray
And you tell me,
Life got in the way!
Then no longer complain
Nor cry when alone"

'But, life got in the way!"

And this dear friend
The one who reads my words
Is not where I wish to see you fall
Into the depth of an illness
Calling loudly for you to hear

So, before the silence beckons
Using screaming as its mode
Step back from life
Provide space for healing
I do not want to hear once more

"But life got in the way!"

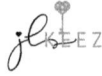

The Orchestra of Life

The piano notes softly speak
The violin when called joins in
The flute gives meaning to the sound

The clarinet in sync steps forth
The guitar riff details the depth of melody
The drums demonstrate strength

The bells in recognition ring
The saxophone delivers the lilt
The keyboard occasioned its tune

The trumpet loudly, gladly played
The cymbal acknowledged its role
The french horn stood proud

The percussion refreshingly breathed
The cello provided backbone
The harp, a sweetness of kind

The viola skipped along expressing joy
The trombone consistently supported
The vocalist completed the beauty

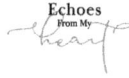

This is the symphony of sound
Unison in presentation
Reflecting the magic, the peace

When in recovery, you
The vocalist
Finds position centre stage

When in recovery, you
The vocalist
Owns position centre stage

The stage which is
Your life

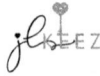

jℓKEEZ

Harp

The strings of the harp
In melodic unity
Whisper my name
Upon sounds of bliss
Heralding, welcoming
The wonder, the powerful
Interwoven blend
Of the one I am
In pure harmony

© 2022 J.L. Keez

The Wind in a Bustle

The wind in a bustle
Whips up the finest of leaves
Sweeps up the purest of flowers
And most vivacious greenery from trees

The wind in a bustle
With expert timing
Combines the leaves
With the flowers
And most vivacious greenery from trees

The wind in a bustle
Although seemingly
Hurried in its pursuit
Knows just how to arrange
The leaves, the flowers
And the most vivacious greenery from the trees

The wind in a bustle
Is simply creating
A wonderful bouquet
Varied yet fine in its look
Colourful yet pure in its character
And most vivacious in its final presentation
A cherished collection

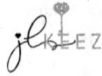

The wind in a bustle
Knows exactly who you are
The finest of souls
The purest of beings
The most vivacious of inspiration
For the wind, ever so watchful
Has observed you for years
And now sees you are ready

To be, to reflect, to give character
To own the leaves
The flowers
And the most vivacious greenery from the trees
For the journey of healing
Now completes
In gratitude, sincerity
We thank
The wind in a bustle

Hum

The humming bird, it hums
In observation I ask why
The humming bird replies
For life is of our doing
If I fly around angry
Anger is what I will attract
If I fly around upset
Tears is what I will attract
If I fly around without looking
Blocks is what I will attract
If I fly around not caring
Most likely enemies is what I will attract

But if I fill my moments
With hums
Or even songs
In certainty I will attract
The peace I do deserve
The happiness I do deserve

To move through life
With freedom
For this is why I hum

© 2022 J.L. Keez

Tween "No" and "Yes"

When the world said "No"
In defiance I said "Yes"
The seemingly insurmountable
For a moment took hold

I stood on that bridge
Tween "No" and "Yes"
Pondering the choice
Laid bare

Is the struggle too much
Is there no way out
Is jumping more attractive
Is there hope enough

All of a sudden
Tween "No" and "Yes"
A vision of me
Wearing a smile presented

Peering deep within the smile
Words joined the vision
I listened, intent
Upon hearing the message

"Tween "No" and "Yes"
Exists your decision
Come closer to see
The choice you are making
Does include me"

So closer I went
And there with the words
My soul now soared
Above the one
Standing upon the bridge

My soul was stunning
Emanating power
In a flash of acknowledgment
The purpose I felt
The choice became clear

Tween "No" and "Yes"
Was a most wonderful place
A destination in reach
Filling with tears
The way moving forward now clear

The soul flying high
Gave the words I required
Words that would tell me
That answers to suffering
Were waiting for me

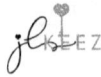

In trust I stepped back
The ledge I vacated
With a smile now smiling
And a body now knowing
In triumph
I strode toward freedom
At the end of the bridge
For there in readiness
Waiting for me
Were the answers long sought

Tween "No" and "Yes"

The Bells of Jubilation

The bells of jubilation
Ring out
The blended tones of recovery
Working together
To deliver the most wondrous
Chime

The bells of jubilation
Sound loud
Shouting to the world
The one who suffered
Has met their liberation
A spirit is free

The bells of jubilation
Chorus in time
To welcome this soul
In revelation
To a life
Renewed by healings hand

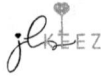

The bells of jubilation
Now quiet
Have heralded the new
The soul, the spirit
In admired gratitude
Now breathes

The kind of breath
That draws in new life
Filled with the strength
Once absent in form
Now present in droves
Applauded in recognition by

The bells of jubilation

Camera

With lightening speed
The camera shuttered
The moment, the instant
Awaited for
Had finally appeared
The glimpse of beauty
Of authenticity
Was finally there to be seen
Where the hand of recovery
Had firmly reached out
Taken hold
And pulled the one
Who suffered
Into triumphant view

The camera had waited patiently
Throughout the years of pain
But knew the day, the time
Would arrive
When in excited jubilation
Its shutter
Would shutter
Capturing the very second
When suffering was no more
And healing, a welcomed
Vision

jLKEEZ

I

I lost my soul
Because of your existence
I lost my heart
Because of your existence
I lost myself
Because of your existence

So where do I go now
Because of your existence
So what do I do now
Because of your existence
So what of my life now
Because of your existence

Well, I find my strength
Because of your existence
Well, I find my happiness
Because of your existence
Well, I turn my trauma
Because of your existence

Into a triumph
Filled with smiles and joy

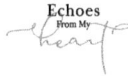

For this is the outcome
Where abuse gave birth
To the wonders of recovery
Where losing me
Turned into
Discovering me

Renewed ... this is what I do!

© 2022 J.L. Keez

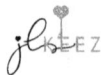

Beauty

Within the fabric of the body
Lies the tapestry of the soul
The content of life lived
Expressed in countless ways

There is colour
Black, white and grey
The texture varies
Smooth, rough, bubbles and spikes

Emotions of life surface, entangled
Soft muffled cries
Smiles in the presence of fun
Despair heard through yelling

Jubilation reflected through song
Grumbles as life twists
Glee laced through the folds
Fear felt like needles jabs

Nostalgia delivers wistful fluffy moments
Anxiety overwhelms changing the design
Boredom splashes pale brown
Calm swirls shades of welcome blue

Anger splinters and splatters red
Confusion threatens to tear
Surprise lifts the soul
Sadness pushes and pulls the threads

Awe sees the tapestry twirl
Emphatic pain shreds
Amusement lightens the load
Admiration mends the rips conveying hope

This is the fabric of the body
The tapestry of expression
Felt by the soul
Where design and life collide

Then there is the final expression
The one we all possess
Where the fabric, the tapestry
In combined agreement

Bring to the surface
Happiness in spades
Joy woven through the layers
Bursts of divine colour

Beauty...

For although the life lived
Influences the fabrics description
And complexion of the tapestry
The soul does carry the strength

jL Keez

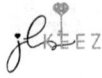

To rise above those inflicting pain
To learn from their existence
Bringing to life
In its own conclusion, its own portrayal

Beauty … colourful, seamless

The Bin!

The riddle of the soul
Perplexing, mysterious
Confuses in its telling

Until with pivotal commitment
The scepticism felt succumbs
To the souls enquiring thoughts

The healing hand of justice
The understanding through honesty
Sends the riddle of the soul

Spiralling, collapsing
With no other place to go
But that extremely useful receptacle

The bin!

Where the epitome of suffering
Is worn by the face
The embodiment of distress
Sees the body droop

Resigned in its demeanour
The owner sheds tears
Which travel down the face
Finding refuge upon the floor

The tears in sad admission
Create puddles in response
The body in confession
Cries out from within

A hand reaches out
A hug delivers warmth
A voice of reassurance
Answers to the call

This is the moment
Where the face, and the body
Sees those tears of admission
Retreat and dry

For in this very instant
The connection between
The epitome of suffering
And the embodiment of distress

Discovers that indeed
There are those who understand
Who will speak the words required
Giving comfort to the call

This my friend
Is where illness finds its end
In the arms of those recovered
The ones who heard your call

Lean on us, learn from us
This is why we arrived
To comfort, guide, inspire
To give our knowledge to you

So the suffering, the distress
Finds its meaning, explanation
Where the face, the body
In renewed acceptance

Softens, stands tall
Ready to live once more
As it was meant
Before life inflicted pain

jLKEEZ

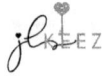

Like a flower opening
To the morning breeze
My heart unfolds
In readiness
To both give
And receive
The sweetness of
Life

Empowerment

The walls of silence
Deafening in their sound
Roar an exacting message

Is this space currently inhabited
Insistent in its position
Enveloping the wounded soul

The only one on offer
Or is there an alternate expression
Awaiting in the wings

Where the chimes of freedom
Ring out in volumed glee
Heralding a prospect yet unknown

Invited investigation may well be
The navigational path to forge
To indeed draw conclusion

The walls of silence
Or, the chimes of freedom
The decision pending

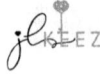

May well see the enveloping lift
The deafening relieved
And the roar disappear

Where chimes fill your day
Glee each moment
And pure understanding

That in owning the prospect
Offered through healing
The heralding, the dawning of

Empowerment
Was there all along
Waiting in the wings

Kindness

The leaf in destination
Floats aimlessly
The breeze
Persuasive in its lead

The addition of sticks
Stones and frogs
Influential in determining
The direction undertaken

Until in recognition
The leaf becomes stuck
Caught between a bottle
And prying fish

Conceding in confession
A more focused, discriminating
Approach is sought
The leaf a little puzzled, groans

Upon reflection
Disgruntlement joins the leaf
In resignation it could now see
The purpose of the obstruction

You see, this leaf
Unaware of others surrounding
Had floated without a care
Without recognition

That choices for existence
Had not held others
In his thoughts
Nor care of repercussion

This instant a consequence
Of selfish venturing
Where decisions had been built
Upon self serving foundations

Now weakened, collapsing followed
A jolt of realisation
A measure of discomfort
Sounding loud throughout his veins

The leaf twists, turns, flips
Desperate to move forward
Attempting to avoid
The bottle and the fish

Escaping found impossible
The leaf a tired mess
Resigned with a breathless
Sigh

Then just like that
A bird descended from above
Pecking at the leaf
A message it did bring

Feeling the pecks of pain
Gasping for air as water engulfs
The leaf now in a tussle
Surrendered to the message

"Shape up, take note
For your actions do inflict
A depth of pain unnoticed
Born from inconsideration"

Visions from the past
Of leaves experiencing tears
Sat the leaf up
The bird, it flew away

Overcome with emotions
Guilt, remorse, repentance
From deep within the veins
A cry for forgiveness rings out

In the absence of kindness
A neglect from childhood learning
This leaf now understands
That where connection exists

Kindness needs to line the
Foundations for life
Where the adjoining framework
Holding the truths for relating

Stands firm, unmoved
Being adopted daily
Into every connection made
Every word spoken

For kindness is the measure
Through which decisions
Choices for life
Must be orchestrated

Upholding, championing
Giving advocacy
To the development of lives
Being absent of struggle

Where kindness underpins
Growth of individuals
Free from mental impairment
Due to societies new understanding

Where compassion accompanies
The seemingly aimless
As each is now armed with
The wisdom

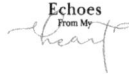

That kindness travels with them
Guides them, fills them
Directing them to be
A companion for others

Where unequivocal acceptance
Dominates the bond
Allowing each to be
Free

Floating without obstruction

© 2022 J.L. Keez

The Door and The Soul

The doors to the soul arched open
A chorus of agony shrilled
Wishing to close the door once more
The soul pulls hard on the handle

Rusty hinges prevent the souls desire
Thus adding to the chorus
Scraping joins the shrill
And together they invade

In vein the soul droops
Realising that closing is impossible
"Then what am I to do"
The soul cries out

The door with caring volume
Responds with words that comfort
"Time has come to investigate
Both the rust and the shrill"

"Let's take this journey together"
Invites the door, "Hold my handle
The adventure ahead will challenge
Guide, yet, inspire"

From that moment forth
In combined confidence
The door and soul become one
The rust dissolved, the shrill left

Now as the door arches open
A chorus of melodic harmonies swirl
The soul in grateful acceptance
Gives thanks to the door

Knowing when arching does occur
Fine tuning is the purpose
So that the rust and shrill
Will no longer hold space

Within the soul

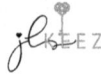

Vision

From the centre of opening blooms
Fragrance floats with ease
Drifting, whirling, gliding

Subsequently resting upon
The leaves of trees
And the soft morning ground

Birds join the scene
Adding sound to the silence
Chirping in rhythmic harmony

Butterflies hover
Hues of magnificent colours
Complete this inspirational stage

The fragrance, the sound, the colours
Reflect the inner joy, the calm, the peace
Of life restored from the depths of misery

This is the vision to have, hold close
An imagination spurring you on
As the road toward recovery invites

Rolling in over the horizon
Clouds took shape with blackened edges
Rain fell hard on the ground below
Sounds thundered louder by the second

In common response I fled
I hid beneath the bed
Yet as I did a voice did ask
"Why are you hiding here?"

Challenged by this thought
Gingerly I crawled from beneath the covers
Slowly opening my eyes
The view inviting, inspiring

Held within awe
The shades of black entwined
The drops of water, grey, the explosion
Spoke deeply to my self

This vision heavenly sent
Reflected the life I had
Blackened, filled with tears
Where emotions thundered

Then, a miracle unfolded
The call to depart was heard
Shining white sparkled, crystal blue appeared,
Silence filled the air

Finding a nearby chair
I sank into its welcome
My mind filled with wonderings
The parallels emerged

My life is like that storm
A blackened rendition lined with grey
Where water wells within my eyes
Releasing emotions deeply confined

So if the storm can find its end
Replaced by the beauty of white, the crispness of blue
Where water disperses, dries
And thunder finds refuge in silence

Surely I can find this too
Where the black of depression
The grey of illness known as mental
The watery tears and deafening despair

Depart

As if to be an after thought
A flash of lightening invaded
Startled, yet not alarmed I understood
This, a moment of striking clarity

The message imposing in its voicing
Was telling me to explore my black
Commune with my tears, hear my despair
To heal from the storm within

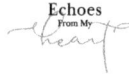

At this very moment a mobile rang
In answering I acknowledged the voice
This was the one sent
To comfort, to guide me through the dark

In response, I said, "Yes"
Readiness, willingness had found me
Clear days were on their way
Inspired by this one

Who had walked the journey before...

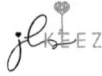

Bell

Bell, I heard you
I mean
Who can escape
The clang of your toll

But bell
I am here to inform you
I am not joining your invite
This time!

To live life in sallowed sanctuary
I am indeed here to release you
From your long
Outstanding service

You see bell
Although you taunt
Although you tease
My strength, my resolve

Finds me able to now rise
Above your clang
In jubilation
To bid you adieu

As I sat beneath the summer sun
Observing the waves of resolution caress the sand
Then retreat in measured determination
The warmth of the morning sun
Evokes, massages, comforts

In response, welcome tears of joy
Find passage from mine eyes
To awaiting hands
In recognition
My mouth smiles, cheeks swell

For this is the moment dreamt
So long ago
Where the path of healing
Met the awareness of
Pain concluding

Where the dawn of life
Renewed by the summer sun
Gave life back to the soul
Once held by suffering's hand
This is the very moment...

As I sit beneath the summer sun

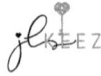

Moments

May I be so bold
To encourage each of you
To live your day
Moment by moment
Moment in moments
Moments in moments in moments

For the more we live by moments
Through moments in moments
We give our full attention
To these glimpses of time
Establishing, building our lives
In reflection

Of Thine

To the tune of the breeze

Beneath the leaves of the trees
Were the birds and the bees
Blissfully playing
To the tune of the breeze

In acknowledged recognition
I wondered why I no longer
Blissfully play
To the tune of the breeze
Beneath the leaves of the trees

Is becoming an adult
Reason enough
To stop blissfully playing
To the tune of the breeze
Beneath the leaves of the trees

In acknowledged recognition
Defiant, I wish to return to
Blissfully play
To the tune of the breeze
Beneath the leaves of the trees

So ... I did!

About the Author

Survivor of a nine-year struggle with anorexia nervosa, and many more enduring associated debilitating, mental illnesses, including chronic fatigue, migraines, anxiety, OCD, depersonalisation and suicidal depression, JL Keez dedicates her life to empowering those impacted as she once was.

A Reality Therapy Certified Counsellor, Speaker and Teacher, J.L. Keez's detailed insights are powerfully portrayed in her first memoir, *Anorexia Unlocked: Understanding Your Story Through Mine*.

JL's second book, *Recovery, and All That Jazz: Mental Illnesses, Life Events and True Understanding* dives deep into the development of mental illnesses, recovery and empowering life moving forward. She particularly highlights the role of relationship(s).

Echoes From My Heart: My words gifted to you to comfort, guide, inspire is purely verse.

Her passionate delivery for The Reality Therapy Institute, Australia, on the topic, "How We Relate ... Impacts" demonstrated her strength as an inspirational voice within her subject area. Speaking for Rotary International, where mental health concerns were discussed, exemplified her gift for presenting.

J.L. Keez educates sufferers of mental illness, with a focus on eating disorders, through educational programs, zoom webinars, inspirational speaking and books. Each medium shared is authentic, honest, highly informative and extremely relatable.

WEBSITE:

jlkeez.com.au

SUBSCRIBE:

J.L. Keez Anorexia Unlocked:
jlkeez.com.au/contact/

FACEBOOK BUSINESS PAGE:

J.L. Keez Anorexia Unlocked:
facebook.com/jlkeez

PRIVATE FACEBOOK GROUP:

Anorexia Unlocked Clients:
facebook.com/groups/jlkeezauc

INSTAGRAM PAGE:

jlkeezanorexiaunlocked:
instagram.com/jlkeezanorexiaunlocked/

LINKEDIN PAGE:

linkedin.com/in/jl-keez-306116203/

CALENDLY BOOKINGS:

https://calendly.com/jlkeez

Acknowledgement

The author recognises the line 'Sunshine, lollypops and rainbows', (pg 81) is the property of the rightful and respective owners:

Composer: Marvin Hamlisch

Vocalist: Lesley Gore, on her 1963 album 'Lesley Gore Sings of Mixed-Up Hearts'.

Arranged by: Claus Ogerman

Produced by: Quincy Jones

www.ingramcontent.com/pod-product-compliance
Lightning Source LLC
Chambersburg PA
CBHW060042030426
42334CB00019B/2454